Hyperthyroidism - The Best Darn Complete Look

Two Popular Hyperthyroid Resources Combined

By: James M. Lowrance © 2013

INTRODUCTION:

This extensive resource, on the subject of hyperthyroidism, contains 18 chapters, with over 14,500 words dedicated to all aspects of hyperthyroid conditions, their symptoms, diagnoses and treatments. I discuss blood and imaging tests and other diagnostic methods for detecting over-functioning thyroid glands, problematic symptoms experienced by "treated hyperthyroid patients" and aspects of improving and optimizing life as a treated thyroid disease patient.

In this resource, I have combined two of my most popular hyperthyroidism eBooks, into one comprehensive resource, at a discounted price.

The content of these combined written works are formatted for easy to follow reading and in language intended for the average layperson thyroid patient. I sincerely believe this resource can benefit hyperthyroid patients, who are seeking to better-understand this metabolic disease that will in the vast majority of cases, require lifelong treatment (hormone replacement, following thyroid removal or ablation).

SECTION ONE

A Complete Look at Hyperthyroidism

Overactive Thyroid Symptoms and Treatments

TABLE OF CONTENTS:

CHAPTER ONE: Hyperthyroidism and Its Causes

CHAPTER TWO: Recognizing Graves' Disease

CHAPTER THREE: Treatments for Grave's Disease

CHAPTER FOUR: Hypothyroid & Hyperthyroid at the Same Time

CHAPTER FIVE: My Own Experience with Hashitoxicosis

CHAPTER SIX: Anxiety Symptoms in Thyroid Disorders

CHAPTER SEVEN: Book Review for: "Living Well with Graves' Disease and Hyperthyroidism"

CHAPTER EIGHT: Goiters Associated with Hyperthyroidism

About the Author:

I am a husband, father, grandfather and lifetime contract salesman, with experience in health writing that began in 2004. I completed theological studies with Liberty University in 1996. I formerly served as editor and forum moderator of Thyroid Health for a major multi-topic content site and as a general health writer for another, where I received Editor's Choice Awards for articles on health subjects.

In 2003 I was diagnosed with hypothyroidism; "Hashimoto's thyroiditis" being the cause. This autoimmune form of thyroid disease that causes destruction of the thyroid gland resulted in my also developing "Chronic Fatigue Syndrome", due to a compromised immune system with severe co-morbid "Adrenal Fatigue". I also suffered severe anxiety symptoms including panic attacks early into the onset of Hashimoto's thyroiditis (Hashitoxicosis–temporary hyperthyroidism).

A common heart murmur I was diagnosed with in my teens called "Mitral Valve Prolapse", also worsened in severity of symptoms with the development of these other health disorders.

Hyperthyroidism - The Best Darn Complete Look

My eventual receiving of diagnoses was a difficult process with proper diagnostic testing not being ordered by the first doctors I sought treatment from. These types of issues were inspiration for me to become proactive in my own health care and to self-educate myself on these health disorders, which I have done extensively since 2003. I now enjoy sharing this information with other patients experiencing my same health disorders.

CHAPTER ONE
Hyperthyroidism and Its Causes

Hyperthyroidism is a term that simply means a person has developed an overactive thyroid gland. The metabolism of a person with hyperthyroidism is sped-up from too much thyroid hormone in their system, so that everything in the body is running at overdrive. When this happens the person will experience hyperthyroid symptoms, which may include the following.

- rapid heart rate
- hyperventilation
- hypertension
- sweating
- inability to sleep
- nervousness and anxiety
- diarrhea
- excessive energy followed by fatigue
- hair loss
- weight loss
- swelling of the thyroid gland (goiter)

Thyroid Autoimmunity

The vast majority of people with hyperthyroidism (95%) experience Graves' disease as the cause. This is an autoimmune disease caused by antibodies created by the immune system that attach to the thyroid gland.

They then begin stimulating it to produce excessive amounts of hormone. The main antibodies responsible for causing Graves' disease are called "Thyroid Stimulating Immunoglobulin" (TSI). When a person has hyperthyroidism, these antibodies are blood tested for to determine whether the cause is from this common autoimmune thyroid disease. They will test positive if the disease is present. Other diagnostic tests for hyperthyroidism may also be performed in addition to a blood draw, to confirm the diagnosis and the cause.

Goiter (Thyroid Gland Swelling)

People with Graves' disease have "toxic diffuse goiters", meaning they have an enlarged thyroid gland that is over-producing. These type goiters are also commonly painful to varied degrees in newly diagnosed Graves' patients. This disease can also have complications and co-morbid conditions associated with it, including one called "Thyroid Eye Disease" (TED – Graves' Ophthalmopathy) an inflammatory condition that can cause severe swelling and bulging of the eyes, plus possible loss of vision if not diagnosed and treated as early as possible (more on this condition in the next chapter).

Hot Nodules

Other possible causes of hyperthyroidism are small tumor-like growths called "thyroid nodules" that can develop in a person's thyroid gland, that begin to absorb iodine and produce thyroid hormones, as if they have become a part of the thyroid gland. These type nodules are called "hot nodules" and are a less common cause of hyperthyroidism but when they do cause thyroid hormone imbalance, it is sometimes referred to as "nodular thyroid disease". Rarely, in some women, tumors on their ovaries can also cause hyperthyroidism as can tumors that occur rarely in the pituitary gland (a master endocrine brain gland).

The "isthmus" (middle portion of the thyroid) is centered in the gland and the two lobes (one on each side) extend upward and are attached to the Adams apple via connecting cartilage (the Adams apple itself is cartilage). It is a butterfly-shaped gland located just below the Adams apple in the front-middle of the neck.

When a goiter (swelling) begins, it can affect only one lobe. A lobe can be affected by a "thyroid nodule" in some cases as well, causing it to protrude on one side of the neck. If both goiter and nodule are present, it may be medically referred to it as a "nodular goiter".

Hyperthyroidism - The Best Darn Complete Look

A doctor can palpate a patient's thyroid gland (feeling with the fingertips) to see if he detects a nodule and whether or not if feels firm/solid. From there he would likely order a thyroid ultrasound and/or a thyroid uptake scan (radioactive iodine dose, followed by radiological imaging), for a more definitive evaluation.

If a thyroid nodule is found and is of a large size or it appears solid, a thyroid tissue biopsy might follow or what is also referred to as a "Fine Needle Aspiration" (FNA) to make sure no cancer cells are present.

If no nodules are found, a patient may simply be experiencing thyroid autoimmunity with resulting inflammation which will eventually lead to hypothyroidism (low functioning thyroid gland) and the goiter may shrink once they are placed on thyroid hormone replacement - once it is needed (some autoimmune hypothyroid conditions may first manifest with a period of hyperthyroidism).

Patients can also experience mild, temporary goiters which can occur with upper respiratory viruses (sub acute thyroiditis), that will resolve over a few weeks period of time. A qualified thyroid doctor can better determine the cause of a swollen thyroid gland or an affected lobe.

In some cases, it may be determined that swelling is not actually within the thyroid but rather within a lymph node located near the gland (e.g. In cases of glandular fever and with types of benign or malignant lymphoma).

Temporary Thyroiditis

While Graves' Disease is considered a type of autoimmune thyroiditis, there are non-autoimmune types of temporary thyroiditis that can also cause periods of hyperthyroidism, before they resolve over several weeks or months. The most common type of temporary thyroiditis that causes hyperthyroidism is "sub-acute thyroiditis". This type is often associated with respiratory viruses that settle in the gland, causing temporary inflammation and a short-term phase of excessive thyroid hormone production.

Iodine Over-supplementation

Medications containing high levels of iodine can result in the patient taking them to experience hyperthyroidism. The same is true of iodine found in over-the-counter supplements that are taken in excess and in products containing high levels of iodized salt. Foods containing seaweed, also referred to as "kelp", can also be a source of excessive iodine intake if they are consumed frequently or in large portions.

At proper intake levels, these supplements and foods can be very healthy for most individuals. It is important to understand what quantities meet the definition for "recommended daily allowances (RDA), as updated by the National Institute of Medicine, in the USA and included on the labels of most over-the-counter products.

Professional Medical Diagnosis and Testing

If you experience some or all of the symptoms listed previously, see your Doctor about being tested for hyperthyroidism. The most common blood test ordered to detect over-activity by the thyroid gland is the "TSH" – Thyroid Stimulating Hormone (the pituitary hormone that reflects thyroid hormone levels). Some Doctors will also order tests of the "T-4 and T-3" thyroid hormone levels if the TSH level is found to be abnormally low. This thyroid regulating hormone decreases with too much thyroid hormone being released in the body and will fall below normal values if hyperthyroidism is present. So, if thyroid hormones are found to be high and/or the TSH level is low, tests for Graves' disease (including TSI antibodies) would likely follow, to determine if it is the cause, as is typically expected.

CHAPTER TWO

Recognizing Graves' Disease

Some statistics estimate that over three million Americans suffer from Graves' disease, with potentially millions of other cases remaining undiagnosed. This thyroid disorder that causes hyperthyroidism is caused by an autoimmune response that medical science is yet to fully understand, in which the immune system sends out antibodies to attack the thyroid gland as previously mentioned.

Graves' disease, hyperthyroidism, is caused by an autoimmune response in the body.

With Graves' disease, these identified antibodies begin to attach to the thyroid gland and in response, the gland produces more thyroid hormone and the levels become too-high for the body's metabolism to function properly.

It is as if the gland is recognizing these invaders as TSH hormone, rather than as enemies to proper hormone regulation. The resulting sped up metabolism is called "hyperthyroidism" or "throtoxicity", with Graves' disease being the most common cause of an over-functioning thyroid gland.

Thyroid Stimulating Immunoglobulin (TSI) can be detected through blood testing.

Patients who develop Graves' disease can have several antibodies directed against their thyroid glands. The antibodies cause gradual destruction of the gland, plus they can cause swelling/goiter from resulting inflammation.

The type of antibody that contributes to the hyper-functioning of the gland, is the TSI antibody, which I have referenced in other subheadings but that I will continue to reference at different points, as we go along. The TSI are the ones that help to better diagnose a hyperthyroid patient as having Graves' disease, when they are medically lab-detected. They are detected in a patient using blood lab testing as previously mentioned but a doctor may also want to test for antibodies called the anti-thyroidperoxidase ("Anti-TPO") and the anti-thyroglobulin("Anti-TG").

All three of these antibodies can be positive in various combinations and to varied degrees in Graves' patients but they will most often be highly-positive for the TSI ones, as the strongest indicator of the disease.

Hyperthyroidism - The Best Darn Complete Look

Graves' disease and other hyperthyroid patients can develop nodules on their thyroid glands that contribute to the over-production of thyroid hormone.

To recap and expand a bit on this subject I would repeat that these nodules are small tumor-like growths, that begin to develop within the thyroid gland. Some of these are what are referred to as "hot nodules", meaning they cause an increase in thyroid hormone production. Not all nodules that develop within a diseased thyroid gland become "hot"; many do not cause the thyroid to become stimulated to over-produce and these type may be referred to as "cold nodules". Some patients who have multiple nodules that are hot may be medically termed as having a "toxic nodular goiter". If the patient simply has thyroid enlargement or goiter that is characteristic of the disease, it is referred to as "toxic diffuse goiter", which is also another term sometimes used for Graves' disease.

The sped up metabolism of Grave's Disease.

A person with hyperthyroidism, caused by Graves' disease, will experience an overactive metabolism resulting in the symptoms listed in CHAPTER ONE. In adding to the previous description for hyper-metabolism, I would add that the abnormally increased energy levels, cause the body to burn fuels that are consumed, at an excessively high rate.

Things such as food, oxygen and water are metabolized very quickly with hyperthyroidism, requiring an increased intake of them to supply the added demand. This can also cause less of the vital nutrients contained within these fuels to be properly absorbed and retained by the body, due to chronic diarrhea that typically occurs.

If not treated, patients with Graves' disease have increased risk for other serious health problems.

The diseases that cause hyperthyroidism – resulting in hyper-metabolism, must be diagnosed and treated if suspected in a patient. If treatment is delayed for lengthy periods of time, serious health problems can develop which may include the following.

- heart disease (i.e. arrhythmias and/or cardiomyopathy)
- organ damage from sustained hypertension
- chronic osteoporosis & myopathy (bone & muscle loss)
- Graves' Ophthalmopathy (GO)

Graves' Ophthalmopathy is an inflammatory problem that can develop within the eyes. The disorder is also called "Thyroid Eye Disease" and can cause serious damage and possible blindness in some patients.

Unfortunately Graves' disease patients who do develop GO may not be able to prevent eye damage even though they are well treated for their hyperthyroidism.

People with hyperthyroid symptoms need to see a licensed physician to have proper testing and diagnosis of the exact cause for their symptoms. If Graves' disease is diagnosed, there are effective treatments to help correct symptoms and any resulting complications. The possible co-morbid conditions (associated disorders) will be further addressed within the following chapter.

CHAPTER THREE

Treatments for Grave's Disease

As previously discussed, Graves' disease (GD) is an autoimmune thyroid disorder that requires treatment by medical professionals. The disease causes the thyroid gland to produce excessive amounts of hormone, causing an over-active metabolism.

The purpose of treatment is to bring thyroid function back to a normal level and so the goal is to reduce the over-activity of the thyroid gland, so that it is operating at a range considered to be within normal limits.

Anti-thyroid medications are used to slow production of thyroid hormones.

The thyroid gland produces mainly the "T-4 and T-3" hormones, but people with GD have an obvious overabundance of them. Patients will be given a trial of an anti-thyroid medication, which is designed to slow down the overactive thyroid so that thyroid hormones fall within normal values. Two of the more common brands of anti-thyroid medications are methimazole (Tapazole) and propylthiouracil (PTU).

19

Can Hyperthyroidism be resolved with Drug Treatment Only?

The answer that follows below, was to a question posted to me by a hyperthyroid patient who was treated with an anti-thyroid drug only (NeoMercazole) and afterward they were placed on thyroid hormone replacement (Eltroxin) for hypothyroidism. It is actually rare for hyperthyroid cases to not require destruction or removal of the thyroid gland and is one of several points I made within my comments to the person who queried me. My response to them, follows. ---

"NeoMercazole is an antithyroid medication that slows thyroid hormone production in an overactive gland. With your hyperthyroidism resolving with this medication and not also requiring thyroid removal, it may have been a rare case in which Graves' disease (autoimmune caused hyperthyroidism) resolved without further treatment. It may also be that your case was actually that of Hashimoto's thyroiditis (a common autoimmune caused hypothyroidism) which can first present with a phase of hyperthyroidism - "Hashitoxicosis".

Your doctor could order tests for Anti-TPO and anti-TG antibodies and if one or both are positive, Hashimoto's would be a strong possibility.

A tissue biopsy called an "FNA" (Fine Needle Aspiration) and a thyroid ultrasound would help confirm this as well, plus the latter one can help detect whether or not any thyroid nodules are present. The type called "hot nodules" can also be a cause of hyperthyroidism.

Eltroxin is a thyroid hormone replacement drug and many Thyroid Specialists and Endocrinologists suggest getting the TSH level (a blood hormone level most often used to monitor thyroid hormone replacement) suppressed down to between "1.0 and 2.0" to better optimized relief of hypothyroid symptoms (like fatigue). Some use "1.0" as their target treatment goal. These are things you might considerdiscussing with your doctor, to better understand your case."

(End of My Reply)

Beta-blocker medications may also be used to control some of the symptoms of hyperthyroidism caused by GD.

Beta-blockers commonly prescribed for high blood pressure, are drugs that block the effects of adrenaline, which is a major hormone sent out by the adrenal glands that helps stimulate heart rate and blood pressure regulation.

Patients with GD may have increased heart rate (tachycardia) and increased blood pressure (hypertension), so administration of a beta-blocker as part of their treatment regimen may sometimes be used to control these abnormally high functioning bodily responses. Some GD patients may only be treated with a beta-blocker or only with an anti-thyroid medication, while some may be treated with both medications simultaneously. This is determined by the severity and types of symptoms being experienced.

Patients who have hyperthyroidism that cannot be controlled well using oral medications may need their thyroid gland surgically removed or destroyed.

When a GD patient or someone with hyperthyroidism from other causes experiences severe symptoms, their doctor may refer them to an Endocrine Surgeon for partial or total removal of their thyroid gland (this is true in most cases). The names for these surgeries are "Total Thyroidectomy"-- meaning an entire gland removal and "Subtotal Thyroidectomy" -- meaning partial gland removal.

In recap for describing the thyroid gland, it is butterfly-shaped and located in the center of the neck, just below the Adams apple.

It has a middle portion called the "isthmus" and a lobe on each side and only some or all of these parts of the gland may need to be surgically removed. Once this surgery has been performed, there is less or none of the thyroid gland in the patient's body to over-produce thyroid hormones. In some cases only one lobe of the thyroid gland is removed (lobectomy), such as when a hot nodule is present or only one side of the gland is affected for other reasons.

Some doctors may want to fully eradicate/remove the gland through a "Radioactive Iodine" treatment, called "thyroid ablation", which is designed to destroy the thyroid gland and completely eradicate it from the body, rather than removing it surgically.

What are the Pros and Cons of RAI Thyroid Gland Ablation?

After corresponding with literally 1,000s of thyroid patients since year-2003, much of this being when I moderated patient-forums, lots of stories were related to me by patients who underwent RAI ablation, who had adverse reactions to it. Some saw a worsening of their thyroid eye disease for example, after weeks post-procedure. Others had successful ablations with no complications. This is why patients referred for the treatment should be thoroughly informed about risks and given the option of surgical thyroidectomy as an alternative choice.

Most of this determination will be made by the treating doctor who is aware of any risks that might be involved with either procedure.

Thyroidectomies also have risks, such as inadvertent damage or removal of the parathyroid glands (those that regulate calcium levels in the body) but if a patient has difficult-to-treat hyperthyroidism, they must undergo one or the other (RAI ablation or surgical removal). As previously stated, if severe hyperthyroidism is allowed to continue, heart problems and severe bone loss can occur. These risks are also why I personally believe patients with milder cases, should first have drug treatment attempted (i.e. anti-thyroid and/or beta-blocker drugs) before thyroid-removal options are offered. This of course depends on the severity of their symptoms and whether or not serious complications have already developed. If drug therapies are not successful, then a choice has to me made between these other two options for gland removal. Lots of endocrinologists and thyroid specializing MDs agree with this opinion.

Anyone seeking information on the subject of thyroid removal, should write down the specific areas of information they are seeking in regard to RAI and/or thyroidectomy and discuss them with their doctor.

Or they can post them on a doctor-moderated forum, that has questions answered by a board certified endocrinologist or thyroid-specializing MD of some type.

Patients who undergo thyroid removal of any type, afterward have no thyroid gland in their bodies and so they become hypothyroid (low thyroid hormone) following removal or ablation. With both types of thyroid removal treatments, the patient will afterward have to be replaced lifelong with the missing hormone, through "Thyroid Hormone Replacement Therapy" (prescribed medication).

The goal of thyroid hormone replacement is to suppress the TSH level (pituitary hormone) and to elevate the T4 and T3 to mid-range or above, following thyroid removal or ablation. A blood TSH level over "10.0" indicates overt (full blown) hypothyroidism but a monitoring doctor might begin hormone replacement sooner. TSH elevates with hypothyroidism, while the thyroid hormones (T4 & T3) decrease to abnormally low levels; the opposite of how hyperthyroid conditions present. The average normal value at blood testing labs for TSH is 0.4 to 4.5 and a thyroid hormone replacement dose will need to get the TSH back down into this normal values range.

Some doctors have a goal of suppressing TSH down to between "1.0 and 2.0" to successfully resolve hypothyroid symptoms of fatigue, weight gain, dry skin, constipation, etc...

Thyroid hormone replacement medications are designed to replace the low level no longer being supplied by the missing or underactive thyroid gland. This condition causes a slowing of the metabolism which means fuels coming into the body (i.e. food and oxygen) are burned/used at a slower than normal rate. By administering thyroid hormone therapy -- dosed to a proper level, the metabolism is brought back up to normal speed for adequate energy levels.

If a proper dose-level is reached but more hormone is added (unnecessary dose increase - over treatment) the metabolism then becomes abnormally sped-up again. This would be referred to as "dose induced thyrotoxicity" (hyperthyroidism from over-supplementation). An overactive thyroid gland or thyrotoxicity from whatever cause (i.e. Graves' disease, thyroid hormone drug or hot nodules in the thyroid gland) will typically cause weight loss as a major symptom. Food passes through the body too quickly for nutrients to be absorbed or for fat to be stored in the body. This is also why diarrhea is a common symptom.

When GD patients develop "Graves' ophthalmology", this will require proper treatment.

Graves' Ophthalmopathy (GO), the previously-mentioned inflammatory condition affecting the eyes, also called Thyroid Eye Disease, can be a complication of Graves' disease in approximately 25 percent of patients. Cases of GO can be mild, moderate or severe and can potentially cause bulging of the eyes and possible deterioration of vision.

The most common treatments for GO include:

• Eye drops to keep the eyes lubricated

• Corticosteroid therapy (steroid anti-inflammatory)

• Radiotherapy and/or Decompression Therapy to reduce orbital damage

• Eyelid surgery, to lengthen eyelids that may not cover the eyes well, due to them bulging.

GD patients who smoke are also encouraged by their doctors to quit smoking because of the inflammatory chemicals contained in cigarettes that can potentially affect the eyes and worsen GO.

CHAPTER FOUR

Hypothyroid & Hyperthyroid at the Same Time

People with another type of thyroid autoimmune disease, that eventually causes progressive hypothyroidism (under active thyroid), called "Hashimoto's thyroiditis", can for a period of time go through phases of hyperthyroidism which is referred to as "Hashitoxicosis". This demonstrates how closely related this condition is to Graves' disease and in-fact these patients may actually transition over to Graves' disease at a later time. While this is not common, it does occur and is something patients need to be aware of if they are experiencing phases that transition back and forth between hypothyroid and hyperthyroid states.

Autoimmune Thyroiditis

With Hashimoto's thyroiditis, which typically causes hypothyroidism (low thyroid hormone) some patients can have fluctuations from hypothyroid to hyperthyroid during the early stage of the disease. This can be due to having high levels of thyroid antibodies. The antibodies that are tested for, when Hashimoto's is being diagnosed are the "TPO" (anti-thyroidperoxidase) and the "TG" (anti-thyroglobulin) antibodies. Either or both testing positive in the blood, helps to confirm the diagnosis.

Some Hashimoto's patients also test positive for the "TSI" antibodies but these are more commonly detected in low titers (low positive), as apposed to high levels found in Grave's patients. Hashimoto's patients who present with high titers of TSI are those who can experience phases of Hashitoxicosis during the early phase of the disease-process.

Thyroid Stimulating Immunoglobulin

The TSI antibody usually contributes to Graves' disease or "autoimmune hyperthyroidism" however, some Hashimoto's patients have these antibodies in addition to the TPO and/or TG ones, causing them to experience spells of Hashitoxicosis or "intermittent hyperthyroidism". This is especially true if at certain points, the antibodies increase to high levels. You could almost say they are suffering from Graves' and Hashimoto's, simultaneously during these phases.

Even without having the TSI antibodies present, Hashimoto's patients can potentially experience flares of thyroiditis, which can also cause mild hyperthyroid type symptoms. These are not usually as severe as those caused by Hashitoxicosis but can still be concerning. Some practitioners within the medical community do not recognize mild Hashitoxicosis but some hypothyroid patients still commonly complain of experiencing spells of mild to moderate hyperthyroid symptoms.

For some of them the hyperthyroid spells can also be due to a spike in thyroid hormone levels from their replacement therapy to correct hypothyroidism, rather than from TSI antibodies being present.

I recently posted on a thyroid forum, in regard to being found in a state of over-treated hypothyroidism. Following is my descriptive post in regard to this issue and how it was resolved by my doctor. ---

"Something has come up in the area of my hypothyroid treatment via Armour thyroid brand, combination - T4/T3 thyroid hormone replacement medication.

You will be blown away when you hear what my recent blood levels of the hormone tested at (via follow-up retests to monitor my dose) because I should be bouncing off the walls with hyperthyroid symptoms. Instead, I'm mainly fatigued, with stressed-out feelings. I do have muscle weakness and have been seeing a neurologist due to a few more sensory and tingling symptoms of aching, occasional stabbing pains etc... I had some low amplitude readings on an EMG but it's possible any nerve damage I have will be helped via the fact I was also found vitamin deficient in D, E and insufficient (low normal) in B12, which are all now being treated.

Now to my blood labs - (ready for this?)---

My TSH result was at "0.05" - Range 0.25 to 5.00 [TSH drops below normal with hyperthyroidism]

My FT3 was a whopping "903" - Range 210 to 440 [elevates with hyperthyroidism]

My Total T3 was nearly as bad (I prefer the Free T3 if only one test is being ordered), which was @ "365" - Range 76 to 181 [also hyperthyroid level]

Yowzah! - Both T3s were more than TWICE the highest normal cut off value! In spite of this, my Dr.s Office called and said my levels were only "a little high" and in fact were going to place me on a DOSE INCREASE prior to seeing these results, because I have gained a little weight since my last visit and my T4 was actually on the low-side, which has been typical of how Armour manifests on my labs for the 7 or 8 years I've been treated with it. It was I who demanded my T3 be tested because they kept failing to add it on my lab requisitions, even with my repeated requests and I had a suspicion the levels were high.

Can a person have these high of levels and not actually feel like metabolism is sped up (hyperthyroid)?

Regardless, I know it is very unwise to maintain this type level due to risk of bone loss and possible heart rhythm complications.

I'm now also beginning to wonder if my high levels of T3 have contributed to my muscle weakness and peripheral neuropathy type symptoms (I know it is not the cause, since I began experiencing these symptoms long before the over-treated thyroid)!

In defense of the doctor, I will say that she had not yet seen the T3 result when she recommended the dose increase but based the idea on my T4 which was at "0.8" in the range of 0.9 to 1.8 ng/dL.

My disappointment with the doctor is in the fact that a former MD I went to, who discontinued his practice due to a back problem, told me that T3 was important to test when taking Armour. I told the new doctor this at my first visit with her back in February, 2010 but she kept failing to add the test on my thyroid panels. I made sure it was added this time, by kicking and screaming a little and sure enough I'm over-treated.

I'm currently taking 2.5 grains, so will reduce it back to 2 grains and hopefully this will be enough of a decrease between now and when I get back in to a doctor."

(**NOTE**: I have conferred with my doctor who agreed with the dose decrease and is monitoring it with follow-up blood retests and my thyrotoxicity is now corrected.)."

The Uncommon Block & Replace Treatment

Some patients who have both Hashimoto's and Graves' antibodies that cause continuously unstable thyroid hormone levels are placed on a treatment called "block and replace". This is a treatment in which they will block the stimulation of the thyroid with an anti-thyroid medication (slows hormone production) and afterward they will replace the patient with thyroid hormone therapy (replaces the diminished hormone levels).

The Rare Transition of Hashimoto's to Graves'

Some Hashimoto's patients have been known to actually transition over to Graves' disease when having both types of antibodies as stated previously and they become progressively hyperthyroid. Other Hashimoto's patients will have hyperthyroid phases but will still become progressively hypothyroid afterward. It may also be encouraging for patients with this condition to know that many Hashimoto's patients have the hyperthyroid spells more-so during the early onset of the disease but after time, the hyperthyroid spells subside and give way to progressive hypothyroidism.

For most hypothyroid patients, their low functioning thyroid state is caused by the autoimmune disease described earlier called "Hashimoto's Thyroiditis".

The disease is characterized by the antibodies previously listed that attack the thyroid gland, due to the immune system mistakenly recognizing it as an enemy in the body that must be destroyed. Usually, the immune system correctly recognizes true invaders and intruders, such as viruses, allergens, fungus and bacteria but in the case of autoimmune disease, the immune system sends antibodies to attack a natural part of the body and commonly this will be the thyroid gland (thyroid autoimmunity).

Dying Thyroid Cells Releasing Stored Hormone

While hashitoxicosis is usually an intermittent condition some medical sources have stated that they believe this condition takes place partly as a result of antibodies that cause the thyroid gland to slowly die off. As previously mentioned, these thyroid antibodies; the main ones being the "anti-Thyroglobulin and anti-ThyroidPeroxidase", are relentless in attacking and eradicating the enemy they have wrongly identified. During this process, thyroid cells do indeed die-off and as they do, any thyroid hormone that is stored within them is released into the bloodstream. Some experts believe this process may contribute to Hashitoxicosis, even when the TSI antibodies are not present.

Normally the thyroid releases these stored hormones, into the blood stream, at a rate that is regulated by the pituitary gland; another master gland, that is found in the brain and the pituitary accomplishes this by means of the regulating hormone - "TSH" (Thyroid Stimulating Hormone), in recap to the previously-discussed. With Hashitoxicosis however, hormone is released at a sporadic rate that is not properly regulated and as a result, the patient experiencing this will have spells of mild Hashitoxicosis despite the fact that they are actually becoming hypothyroid.

These spurts of released thyroid hormone may also be the thyroid gland attempting to fight off the autoimmune attack, in attempt to delay or prevent its own eventual death from the relentless antibodies attack.

These surges of extra hormone actually cause these rapid but short-lived spells of hyperthyroidism however, in some patients with highly elevated thyroid antibody levels these Hashitoxicosis spells may occur more frequently.

This is especially true in earlier stages of the disease and may seem like ongoing hyperthyroidism to the patient and their doctor, who may at-first believe they are manifesting Graves' rather than Hashimoto's disease.

Most Patients Present with Only One Disease

While it is true that some patients with Hashimoto's Thyroiditis may also have co-existing Graves' disease antibodies (TSI), the majority of patients have only one disease or the other. When a patient does have Grave's antibodies co-existing with Hashimoto's antibodies, it may eventually develop into overt hyperthyroidism however, if it is a patient with only the antibodies causing Hashimoto's, their intermittent spells of hyperthyroidism, are likely caused by Hashitoxicosis and not by co-existing Graves' Disease.

Most patients have less frequent spells of Hashitoxicosis over time, as overt hypothyroidism sets in and much of the thyroid gland cells have already died-off but when a patient is experiencing this phenomenon, it can cause unpleasant and concerning symptoms.

Hashitoxicosis and Blood Retesting Thyroid Hormone Levels

It is likely better for a hypothyroid patient to reschedule a blood test follow-up, if they are being monitored for thyroid hormone replacement treatment but are going through a spell of Hashitoxicosis at the time of their blood draw appointment.

Some medical opinions state that Hashitoxicosis will not affect blood tests results to a significant degree, while others believe it can cause results that show a falsely high reading on them, resulting in an incorrect evaluation of treatment hormone levels.

Some medical resources state that Hashitoxicosis is rare however I feel that "mild" cases are likely very common and as a Hashimoto's patient, I experienced intermittent spells of hyperthyroid symptoms early into my own autoimmune hypothyroid disease.

Patients who believe they may be experiencing this medical phenomenon should inform their Doctor and this is especially true if the symptoms seem to be severe and ongoing rather than mild and intermittent.

CHAPTER FIVE

My Own Experience with Hashitoxicosis

I previously described Hashitoxicosis and its relationship to autoimmune hypothyroidism. I also described a point in time in-which I was over-treated with thyroid hormone replacement therapy, which caused me a period of throtoxicosis/thyrotoxicity, which was corrected by my doctor. In this chapter I want to relate my own experience with Hashitoxicosis plus share some additional opinions I have in regard to this intermittent hyperthyroid condition that can happen to patients with Hashimoto's thyroiditis.

When I began suffering thyroid disease symptoms in late year-2002, many of them were classic hypothyroidism symptoms. In addition to these however, I was also experiencing alternating spells of hyperthyroid symptoms. At times these two different sets of symptoms would rapid cycle from one to the other.

Mild Hashitoxicosis more Common than Full-blown

Some Doctors may state that Hashitoxicosis can only be identified as such, if the hyperthyroid symptoms are severe however I believe that Hashitoxicosis can occur more commonly in milder forms.

Just like there can be cases of sub-clinical Graves' disease (hyperthyroidism), I believe patients can also experience sub-clinical spells of Hashitoxicosis. It might be a better term to refer to these less-severe hyper spells as simply "thyroiditis flares" but regardless of the term used, these spells or phases result in mild to moderate symptoms of hyperthyroidism.

My Hashitoxicosis or "hypothyroid cycling with hyperthyroid" would happen more often at night when I was trying to fall asleep and in the mornings upon waking but at other times, it would manifest anytime during the day as well. My thought patterns had nothing to do with these hyperthyroid spells and I knew for a fact that it was not a result of typical anxiety. I also do not experience sweating with anxiety and never had previous to thyroid disease but with these hyperthyroid spells I would sweat profusely and I would soak the bed I was laying on.

During several weeks of this hyper-phase cycling, I lost eight pounds of weight (I wish I had kept it off) but once these more severe hyperthyroid spells subsided, I became progressively hypothyroid. While I still have mild hyper phases from time to time, they are much farther between and are less severe.

These can likely be attributable to mild fluctuations in my thyroid hormone replacement therapy levels, which can be mildly affected by things such as diet and a change in my level of physical activity.

Throiditis Flares versus Hashitoxicosis

I do still have the occasional mild spells of Hashitoxicosis or what might actually be better termed as "thyroiditis flares". Recently, my Doctor reviewed some blood retests I had done over an approximate six month period to monitor my hormone replacement therapy. There were clearly times I was borderline hyperthyroid and even slightly flagged-high on my dose of thyroid hormone replacement, while on previous and succeeding tests I was only about mid-range or slightly above on my thyroid hormone levels. This was while taking the **same dose** of thyroid hormone medication. The fact is, some treated hypothyroid patients stay leveled-out on their thyroid dose better than others do and this can be a result of varying degrees of Hashitoxicosis/thyroiditis flares in my opinion. Mild Hashitoxicosis or if you prefer to call it thyroiditis flares, are possibly more common than some medical sources may believe them to be and this may also be a factor in explaining why some Hashimoto's patients struggle more than others do, with ongoing anxiety symptoms. More on the anxiety aspect of hyperthyroidism will be discussed in CHAPTER SIX.

My Advice to a Patient with both Hyperthyroid and Hypothyroid Symptoms

I was talking to a woman who visited her Doctor due to symptoms she was having of unusual weight gain and fatigue, which are usually associated with being hypothyroid but some of her symptoms were more indicative of a hyperthyroid condition. Her Doctor immediately pronounced her as having depression but she felt within her body that further investigation of her symptoms was merited. Upon her Doctor ordering her tests for "thyroid antibodies" and of her TSH level (which she had to request), both came back abnormal. Her TSH being flagged below-normal indicated an overactive thyroid gland.

Her thyroid antibodies tested positive and were flagged hundreds of points above normal, indicating autoimmune thyroid disease. Her symptoms however were those of hypothyroidism or an under-active thyroid. I pointed out to her the fact that the two diseases (Hashimoto's and Graves') can cause positive thyroid antibodies but I also pointed out how these two diseases can have crossover-symptoms early into the onset of them. Her case, like many thyroid disease patients was in need of further investigation by a qualified physician.

This was the Basic Advice I Related to Her

QUOTE:*"Your story is typical and unfortunately I hear it so often, it is alarming. Your choice to see an Endocrinologist is a wise one and I'm willing to bet you'll get proper testing and treatment from him/her.*

There are two possibilities with your thyroid antibodies being highly-elevated and that would be that you either have "Hashimoto's thyroiditis" (autoimmune hypothyroidism) or "Graves' disease" (autoimmune hyperthyroidism). I lean toward Hashimoto's because that was likely the TPO (anti-thyroidperoxidase) test you had a high-positive result on and it is highly elevated more often in Hashimoto's than in Graves'. The "TSI" antibody is one more typical of Graves' "Thyroid Stimulating Imunnoglobulin" but can be present in Hashimoto's as well and will cause hyperthyroid phases (Hashitoxicosis) before it causes progressive hypothyroidism.

My suspicion is that your Endocrinologist will want to test you for the TSI antibodies as well, if your TSH is still low. He will also likely want to test your T-3 and T-4 thyroid hormone levels. He will likely also palpate your thyroid (feel with fingertips) to see if you have palpable (detectable) goiter (general thyroid swelling) or nodules (growth-tumors).

If any are found, he may want to send you for a thyroid ultrasound, which will give detailed imaging of your thyroid. Some patients with autoimmune thyroid disease have "hot nodules" that actually cause the thyroid gland to produce too much hormone.

It sounds like, with highly elevated antibodies and a flagged-low TSH on two consecutive tests, your case needs further investigation. I commend you for demanding those tests that led them on the right track, rather than accepting the emotional diagnosis. Your story in that regard is very similar to mine and many other thyroid patients I have corresponded with." END QUOTE

CHAPTER SIX

Anxiety Symptoms in Thyroid Disorders

Anxiety symptoms are one possible manifestation of hyperthyroidism or an over-active thyroid gland but they can also occur in people with hypothyroidism. Patients with thyroid disorders commonly report the following anxiety symptoms.

- nervousness
- feeling on edge
- panic attacks
- free-floating anxiety symptoms (generalized anxiety)

When a patient visits their Doctor with these symptoms combined with other hyperthyroid symptoms such as excessive energy, weight loss, hair loss, sweating, diarrhea and swelling or pain in their thyroid, blood tests of thyroid function should be ordered.

This is true even if only one or two of these symptoms are present. Basics about diagnosis and treatment of hyperthyroidism will be mentioned again in the following subheadings but bears repeating as related to resolving symptoms of anxiety.

Slowing Down the Thyroid and Addressing Symptoms

If a patient is found to have hyperthyroidism, the treatment would be to slow down the thyroid by use of oral medications. These medications are called "Anti-Thyroid Medications", which slow down the thyroid's overproduction of thyroid hormone, as previously discussed. Patients may also be given beta-blockers, which are medications designed to block the effects of the over-production of adrenaline experienced by hyperthyroid patients. In both cases, the results can be a decrease in chronic anxiety and/or panic symptoms that are being experienced.

Gland Removal or Ablation

In more severe cases of hyperthyroidism, the thyroid may be partially or completely removed through surgery or the gland may be partially destroyed through Radioactive Iodine treatment (RAI). With RAI, also called "Ablation", they give the patient a solution of iodine, that is radioactive and it will go directly to the thyroid gland, destroying thyroid cells, resulting in slowing down its overproduction of thyroid hormones. Following this procedure, the over-active metabolism, that can contribute to anxiety symptoms, is slowed, which helps them to diminish.

Hypothyroid Therapy

Once a hyperthyroid patient is treated via gland removal or ablation, they will then become hypothyroid and require that it be treated. The treatment for hypothyroidism is also by oral medication but in this case, medications called "Thyroid Hormone Replacement Medications" are used to supplement the thyroid's inadequate, underproduction of thyroid hormones.

The most common method used to diagnose thyroid disorders, is through blood testing. Blood is drawn and lab-tested to see if the thyroid's hormone levels are in the normal range. If they are outside of the normal reference range, on the high end, this would indicate an over-active thyroid gland, "hyperthyroidism". If the hormone levels are found to be outside of the range on the low end, it would indicate an under-active thyroid gland, "hypothyroidism" and hormone replacement therapy would be needed.

TSH – The Most Sensitive Thyroid Function Test

In adding a bit more to the previous discussion on TSH, I would add that it is the most sensitive thyroid function test available. It is the one that many Doctors will use alone before testing the actual thyroid hormones.

As mentioned previously, it is not actually a thyroid hormone but one that comes from the "pituitary gland" (brain gland). This gland regulates the thyroid by means of TSH, which it sends to the thyroid, stimulating it into producing its own hormones at the proper levels.

If TSH is found to be low, this would indicate that the thyroid gland is no longer being stimulated by the pituitary to produce hormones because it is already over-active. If TSH is found to be high, this would indicate that the pituitary is working too-hard to get the thyroid to produce hormones because it is under-active. So TSH is a valuable test because of its sensitivity in monitoring thyroid function.

If you suspect you have thyroid disease, that is either causing or aggravating your anxiety symptoms or if you experience some of the other symptoms that indicate possible thyroid dysfunction, talk to your Doctor about getting your TSH tested because if hyperthyroidism or thyroid autoimmunity is the cause, treatment will go a long way toward relieving these symptoms of chronic anxiousness.

CHAPTER SEVEN

Book Review for: "Living Well with Graves' Disease and Hyperthyroidism"

As a Thyroid Patient Advocate, I am inspired to share other helpful resources with fellow thyroid patients. Another Thyroid Patient Advocate who has done a great deal for patient-education and in providing resources to help thyroid patients to become proactive in their treatments, is Mary Shomon. She has been in the advocacy arena for a number of years longer than I have, her diagnosis of thyroid disease preceding mine by several years as well.

She has bestowed me the honor of reviewing a number of her books, including the one I will address in this chapter. She was kind enough to send me a free copy for reviewing and this is my review of this wonderful book on the subject of hyperthyroidism and Graves' disease.

Mary Shomon's book "Living Well with Graves' Disease and Hyperthyroidism" is a complete and thorough resource to help educate patients being treated for overactive thyroid glands of all causes, including Graves' Disease, which is the number one cause of hyperthyroidism worldwide.

I appreciate the fact that Mary authored a book specifically for hyperthyroid patients and others who wish to learn about this thyroid disease, rather than simply including a detailed section for it in one of her other thyroid subject books. She could have easily done this with the fact that hypothyroid (under active thyroid) patients outnumber those with hyperthyroid conditions by about five to one. I believe this demonstrates her passion for providing thorough, quality information for hyperthyroid patients who also wish to live well with their disease. This book helps these patients to achieve this and to gain back as much quality-of-life as possible as treated hyperthyroid patients.

She addresses in detail the signs and symptoms of hyperthyroidism, including those physical ones caused by an abnormally increased metabolism in the body. She also addresses those signs of bodily changes, including goiter (thyroid swelling), nodules (tumors on/in the gland), hair loss and weight loss as well as the emotional symptoms of anxiety and depression. Co-morbid conditions caused by hyperthyroidism and Graves' are also discussed, including eye inflammation (Graves' Ophthalmopathy) and skin related problems (Graves' Dermopathy).

She continues with a chapter on the vastly important subject of getting diagnosed so that treatment for relieving symptoms and to begin healing in the body can be administered by a qualified Doctor. A chapter on integrative and holistic treatments is also included in addition to discussions on conventional medical treatments.

Mary also takes a detailed look at the medical tests used to diagnose hyperthyroid conditions, including common blood tests of thyroid hormone levels and imaging tests that detect toxic goiter and hot nodules that may contribute to overproduction of hormone by the thyroid gland. She also discusses the subject of "thyroid antibodies" with special emphasis on the auto-antibody most commonly associated with Grave's called "Thyroid Stimulating Immunoglobulin" (TSI).

In her thoroughness in covering these subjects related to hyperthyroidism, she also covers aspects relating to breastfeeding, infants, children and teens who, are affected. Also covered is the subject of post treatment hypothyroidism (low thyroid hormone following correction of hyperthyroidism) that requires treatment with thyroid hormone replacement therapy following removal or destruction of the gland in patients who require these type treatments.

I highly recommend this wonderful book to my fellow thyroid patients who suffer hyperthyroidism, to those who suspect they may have an overactive thyroid and to anyone who is simply interested in a detailed study on all the important aspects of this serious but treatable thyroid condition. Patients can in fact live well with this disease and Mary Shomon has provided a great resource in helping patients to achieve this goal. The book is available through major book sellers and I recommend it as another great source for hyperthyroid patients.

CHAPTER EIGHT

Goiters Associated with Hyperthyroidism

In this chapter, I will discuss the subject of "goiters" a bit more because they are a major aspect and manifestation of hyperthyroidism. While I will again describe the more common type goiter found in hyperthyroid patients, I will describe other goiters that can also occur in hyperthyroid patients and in those with thyroid diseases of other kinds. I will repeat some information but will add other aspects not previously covered.

When a thyroid patient has a goiter, this simply means they have swelling of the thyroid gland, which is located at the front of the neck, in the area just below the Adam's apple. Goiters are recognized as different types and as affecting part of the thyroid, such as one of the two lobes or the middle part of the gland called the isthmus or as affecting the entire gland as a whole. They are also considered different types depending upon the causes of them. A major cause of goiters, is thyroid autoimmunity.

Types of Goiters

If a goiter is caused by iodine deficiency, it is referred to as a "colloid nodular" or "endemic" goiter. This type is rare in the U.S. and in most other industrialized countries that use iodized table salt.

Table salt, usually provides those that consume it, enough iodine to avoid iodine deficiency hypothyroidism and the resulting endemic goiters.

If a person's thyroid gland has swelling plus a number of small tumors called "nodules" within it, they refer to this type as a "multi-nodular goiter". The nodules within a gland that has goiter can be the type that causes the thyroid gland to produce excessive thyroid hormone (hyperthyroidism), in which case, they will add the term "toxic" to the term, calling it a "toxic multi-nodular goiter". People with Hashimoto's thyroiditis, commonly have multi-nodular goiters that are non-toxic.

When a person is termed as having a "diffuse goiter", this means there is general swelling throughout the gland that is not caused by nodules. This type of goiter can also cause toxicity or over-activity of the thyroid gland (hyperthyroidism), in which case it is referred to as a "toxic diffuse goiter". These types are found commonly in patients with Graves' disease, as are toxic multi-nodular goiters.

Types of Thyroiditis

Temporary types of thyroiditis, such as those that occur with viral infections and in pregnant women can also cause goiter (asymmetrical enlargement).

These type will resolve within a few weeks, along with the thyroiditis. These type goiters can flare short term with these types of thyroiditis and cause severe pain in the thyroid gland, which is referred to as "subacute thyroiditis", while other types do not cause a painful thyroid which is referred to as "silent thyroiditis". Temporary types of thyroiditis commonly first manifest with a spell of hyperthyroidism.

The Size of a Goiter can Determine its Treatment

A goiter can be mild, so that it is barely visible by looking at the affected person's neck or sometimes not visible at all with the naked eye. The same is true of detecting a goiter by human feel or what they refer to as "palpation". Some cannot be felt or seen but may still have enough swelling present within them, to cause mild discomfort and a mild feeling of inflammation in the neck.

When goiters become severe, they can become large enough to obstruct swallowing and breathing and in these cases, thyroid removal (total-thyroidectomy) might be an option a treating Doctor would consider. When goiters are less severe, treating any thyroid hormone imbalance that is present in the patient can help to shrink them and prevent further growth of them.

Imaging Tests

Patients, who have goiters or who are suspected of having them, may be referred for a "thyroid ultrasound" (sound-wave imaging/sonogram) or "thyroid uptake scan" (radiology/radioactive iodine) and possibly even an MRI (Magnetic Resonance Imaging). These are diagnostic tests that give detailed images of the thyroid gland, to determine the size of goiters and whether they contain nodules within them that are not detectable by palpation.

Self-Monitoring for Symptoms and Reporting to a Doctor

If you feel tightness or swelling in your throat in the area of the thyroid gland, or can actually see visible swelling, report to your Doctor for a checkup and evaluation of your symptoms, making sure to list any other symptoms you are experiencing, in detail. Most goiters can be treated, so that any symptoms they are causing are improved or significantly relieved.

These are general overviews of some of the more common treatments for hyperthyroidism and Graves' disease. Patients with these diseases must be evaluated by qualified, licensed physicians, so that treatment is tailored to each patient individually.

(END – SECTION ONE)

SECTION TWO

The Best Darn Hyperthyroidism Book!

Studies in the Overactive Thyroid Gland

TABLE OF CONTENTS:

<u>CHAPTER ONE</u>:
Hyperthyroidism Basic Facts
Overactive Thyroid Gland General Information
<u>CHAPTER TWO</u>:
Major Causes of Hyperthyroidism and Treatments
Common Contributors to Thyrotoxicity
<u>CHAPTER THREE</u>:
Graves' Disease Hyperthyroidism and Treatments
Autoimmune Caused Hyperthyroidism
<u>CHAPTER FOUR</u>:
Radioactive Iodine Ablation of the Thyroid
Cell Destruction of Diseased Glands
<u>CHAPTER FIVE</u>:
Treatment for Hashitoxicosis versus Graves' Disease
Patients with Temporary Hyperthyroidism
<u>CHAPTER SIX</u>:
Why Doctors Sometimes Delay Treatment for Hashimoto's Thyroiditis
Problems with Hashitoxicosis
<u>CHAPTER SEVEN</u>:
Manifestations of Thyroid Eye Disease
Autoimmune Eyeball Problems and Their Treatments
<u>CHAPTER EIGHT</u>:
Symptoms and Manifestations of Thyroid Storm
The Hyperthyroid condition requiring Emergency Care

Hyperthyroidism - The Best Darn Complete Look

CHAPTER NINE:
Support for Struggling Thyroid Patients
Two Reasons Why Information and Support Resources are Important
CHAPTER TEN:
Coping with Thyroid Disease
Methods for Dealing with a Lifetime Health Disorder

CHAPTER ONE

Hyperthyroidism Basic Facts

Overactive Thyroid Gland General Information

Hyperthyroid disorders account for approximately 20% of thyroid disorder cases. An overactive thyroid gland can cause an array of symptoms but treatments are available.

Hyperthyroidism is a term meaning a person's bodily metabolism is abnormally sped up due to the T3 and/or T4 thyroid hormone levels increasing too high in the body. Symptoms vary in severity among individuals, according to how advanced hyperthyroidism has become at the time of diagnosis.

Major Causes of Hyperthyroidis

Most cases of hyperthyroidism are caused by Graves' disease, the autoimmune disease of the thyroid gland in which auto-antibodies sent from the immune system cause stimulation of excessive amounts of thyroid hormone production. Graves' patients experience thyroid gland inflammation and enlargement to varied degrees, referred to as "toxic diffuse goiters".

Thyroid autoimmunity is a "primary" cause of an overactive thyroid gland.

Another primary cause of an overactive thyroid gland would include "hot nodules", which are tumorous-growths in the gland that absorb iodine in the body and begin producing thyroid hormone just as normal thyroid tissue does.

Less common "secondary" causes of hyperthyroidism include excessive intake of iodine which can also act as a trigger for primary thyroid autoimmunity. Temporary types, of thyroiditis occurring in pregnant women or following giving birth or as a result of viral illnesses that settle in the thyroid gland, will cause a short-term phase of hyperthyroidism. Treated hypothyroid patients can become hyperthyroid from taking too high a dose of thyroid hormone replacement, sometimes referred to as "dose induced thyrotoxicity".

Hyperthyroid Symptoms

The symptoms of a sped up metabolism from hyperthyroidism include:

- nervousness and anxiety
- tremor (especially in the hands)
- rapid pulse and breathing

- hypertension
- diarrhea
- oily skin and hair
- increased sweating
- increased hunger and thirst
- changes in menstrual cycle and sex drive
- goiter
- rapid weight loss

Patients with Graves' disease may also experience symptoms of muscle weakness and wasting referred to as "myopathy". They may also develop an inflammatory condition affecting the eyes called "Graves' Ophthalmopathy" or "Thyroid Eye Disease".

Diagnosis

Blood tests of thyroid hormone levels and/or the TSH level can help to diagnose hyperthyroidism. Thyroid hormones (T4 and T3) will elevate to levels above normal values, while TSH (pituitary hormone) will decrease to levels below normal values. When testing is conducted to determine the cause of hyperthyroidism, blood tests for thyroid antibodies may be ordered to confirm or rule out Graves' disease as the cause.

A Radioactive Iodine Uptake Test (RAIU) might also be performed to determine if the thyroid gland is absorbing high levels of iodine which can indicate that it is overactive. If only a certain area of the gland is absorbing high levels of iodine, this can point to hot nodules and an additional Radioactive Iodine Scan (radiology camera) might also be performed at the same time or separately to further evaluate nodules in the gland.

Treatment

In some cases of hyperthyroidism, the administering of anti-thyroid drugs designed to slow thyroid hormone production will be the initial treatment and possible the only one needed. Beta-blocker medications that moderate the activity of adrenaline in the body can help to alleviate symptoms and may be combined with anti-thyroid drugs.

Surgical procedures are required in some cases of hot nodules, to remove them or part of the thyroid gland if multi-nodules are present (several). Thyroid removal surgery called "thyroidectomy" may also be needed in cases of Graves' disease that cannot be controlled by drug therapies.

The gland may also be ablated (destroyed) through administering radioactive iodine in a large enough to dose to kill-out the entire gland.

Afterward, patients whose thyroid glands are ablated or removed will require thyroid hormone replacement to treat resulting hypothyroidism, as a lifelong treatment.

CHAPTER TWO

Major Causes of Hyperthyroidism and Treatments

Common Contributors to Thyrotoxicity

As mentioned previously, approximately 20% of thyroid disease cases are hyperthyroid conditions. There are several causes for overactive thyroid disorders and treatments available for them.

The term "thyrotoxicity" simply means that abnormally high levels of thyroid hormone in the body are causing a toxic reaction also referred to as "hyperthyroidism". While the majority of hyperthyroid conditions are a result of auto-antibodies that stimulate excessive thyroid hormone levels, there are a number of other causes as addressed in the subheadings that follow.

Temporary Thyroiditis

Some people experiencing viral infections or pregnancies will have a resulting inflammatory reaction in their thyroid glands called "thyroiditis".

Some cases manifest with a painful thyroid gland (sub-acute) while others do not (silent) but the majority of temporary thyroiditis conditions start with a phase of hyperthyroidism. Treatment for high levels of thyroid hormone is usually not necessary since the condition will resolve on its own over several weeks period of time. Treatment may only require bed rest and anti-inflammatory drugs for fever and thyroid inflammation.

Over-consumption of Iodine

People taking drugs that contain high-iodine content or who consume an excessive amount of iodine-rich foods such as kelp (seaweed) or supplements that contain higher-than-recommended daily allowances of iodine can cause hyperthyroidism to be induced.

In these cases, if the excessive iodine intake does not trigger an autoimmune response, causing permanent hyperthyroidism, the treatment would simply be to discontinue use of the products containing high levels of iodine.

Hot Nodules

Thyroid nodules are tumor-like growths that can develop within the thyroid gland. The majority of them do not affect thyroid hormone levels but a small percent can present as "hot nodules". This means the nodule has taken on features similar to thyroid gland tissue and is absorbing iodine coming into the body and producing thyroid hormones from it. This adds more thyroid hormone production to what the gland is already normally producing, causing the levels to become abnormally high.

Treatment for hot nodules may include surgical removal of them or removal of part of the thyroid gland (partial or sub-total thyroidectomy or lobectomy) or of the entire gland (total thyroidectomy). Once thyroid tissue is removed via a corrective procedure, thyroid hormone replacement may also become necessary afterward, as a life long treatment.

Over-treated Hypothyroidism

Thyroid hormone replacement therapy is administered by an oral dose of T4 or combination T4 and T3 prescription thyroid hormone medication.

The dose is then monitored through follow-up blood retests of the hormone levels in the patient's body. If a dose is too high and over-replacement is occurring, medication-induced thyrotoxicity can occur. The treatment would be to reduce the patient's dose and to possibly stop the dose temporarily so that their thyroid hormone levels decrease back down into the normal values range. Afterward the corrected dose-level would also need to be monitored via blood retests and at reasonable intervals throughout the patient's life.

Thyroid Autoimmunity

Graves' disease is the autoimmune cause of progressive hyperthyroidism in which auto-antibodies stimulate excessive production of thyroid hormones. Hashitoxicosis is also an autoimmune cause of hyperthyroidism but in this case, patients with Hashimoto's thyroiditis that typically causes progressive hypothyroidism (under-active) will first see the condition manifest with a phase of temporary hyperthyroidism.

Most patients experiencing Hashitoxicosis will not have additional flares of the condition once it initially resolves.

However, some do experience milder fluctuations in thyroid hormones due to flares of thyroiditis (phases of increased inflammation). In rare cases, Hashimoto's thyroiditis will transition over to Graves' disease but most patients remain hypothyroid and require life-long thyroid hormone replacement therapy.

Treatment for cases of hyperthyroidism from Graves' disease may include anti-thyroid drugs to reduce elevated thyroid hormone levels, beta-blocker medications to reduce hyperthyroid symptoms and possible eventual thyroid removal by surgery (thyroidectomy) or destruction of the gland by radioactive iodine (ablation).

CHAPTER THREE

Graves' Disease Hyperthyroidism and Treatments

Autoimmune Caused Hyperthyroidism

As mentioned in a previous chapter, Graves' disease is the leading cause of hyperthyroidism. Complications can include hypertension, cardiac arrhythmias and thyroid eye disease but treatments are available.

Graves' disease is an autoimmune condition affecting the thyroid gland that results in abnormally high levels of thyroid hormone to be released into the body causing hyperthyroidism. There is no cure for Graves' but progression of the disease can be halted by removing the thyroid gland. Mild to moderate cases may be successfully treated through drug therapies.

How Common is Graves' Disease?

Graves' disease affects up to 1% of the U.S. population or up to 3-million people, which is about 5 in every 10,000 people and is 7 times more common in women than in men.

Graves' patients are among the 190 million people worldwide who experience goiters but in the case of Graves' the goiter is "toxic" (toxic diffuse goiter), meaning it is causing abnormally high thyroid hormone levels or "thyrotoxicity" (hyperthyroidism).

Graves' patients can experience complications from the disease, including an inflammatory condition in the eyes called "Thyroid Eye Disease" or "Graves' Ophthalmology". It is estimated that about half (50%) of all Graves' patient will develop this complication of the disease affecting the eyes.

Is Hyperthyroidism Present in all Graves' Patients?

The point at which hyperthyroidism sets in varies among those found to have the auto-antibodies causing Graves' disease, called "Thyroid Stimulating Immunglobuins" (TSI). Most patients may be positive for these "thyroid antibodies" months or years before the level of them becomes elevated enough to cause hyperthyroidism. The reason this may be the case is due to the fact that most people who are found to have Graves', are tested because they are already manifesting the signs or symptoms of hyperthyroidism.

There are cases in which Graves' patients experience mild, early-onset goiters before their thyroid hormone levels become abnormally high.

Thyroid Antibodies common to both Graves' and Hashimoto's

The TSI are not the only antibodies present with Graves' but will co-exist with other thyroid antibodies that cause thyroid cell destruction, including the anti-thyroidperoxidase (Anti-TPO) and/or the anti-thyroglobulin (Anti-TG). These latter two mentioned antibodies are also present in Hashimoto's thyroiditis (autoimmune hypothyroidism) patients but are usually found in lower titers (positive lab measurements) in Graves' patients.

Some Hashimoto's patients in fact are also found to be positive for TSI antibodies that typically cause Graves' but are in lower titers and may cause temporary hyperthyroid phases (Hashitoxicosis). These facts demonstrate how closely related these two autoimmune thyroid diseases are. It also offers explanation as to why some Graves' patients transition to Hashimoto's over time and the reverse has also been known to happen, although not common.

Symptoms and Treatment for Graves' Hyperthyroidism

When thyroid hormone levels have become abnormally high, causing the body's metabolism to become sped up, hyperthyroidism symptoms will develop. These include increased energy, nervousness and anxiety, rapid heart rate, hypertension, excessive sweating, diarrhea and weight loss. If Thyroid Eye Disease develops, the additional symptoms may include bulging, dryness, double vision (diplopia), and irritation of the eyeballs.

Some cases of Graves'-caused hyperthyroidism are successfully treated with anti-thyroid drugs, which block thyroid hormone, reducing the amount entering the cells of the body and/or beta-blockers, which block the effects of epinephrine (adrenaline). When epinephrine is elevated in the body, it can cause cardiac arrhythmias and hypertension and elevated thyroid hormone levels speed up all bodily functions as a whole.

Determining which drug is needed or if a combination of them is needed, depends on how severe the hyperthyroidism is.

Severe cases of Graves' hyperthyroidism that cannot be successfully treated with drug therapies may require surgical removal of the gland (thyroidectomy) or destruction of the gland using radioactive iodine (ablation). Afterward, patients will need thyroid hormone levels corrected with replacement therapy.

Treatment for Graves' Ophthalmology (Thyroid Eye Disease)

Thyroid Eye Disease (TED) is often treated using anti-inflammatory steroids (corticosteroids) to reduce inflammation, such as Prednisone. Eye drops may also be prescribed to keep dry eyes moistened. In cases when the disease is causing significant pressure on the optic nerve and presents the danger of vision loss, eye surgeries called "orbital radiotherapy" and/or "orbital decompression" may be necessary.

If eye protrusion is causing inability for a patient to close their eyes, surgery may be required to lengthen their eyelids. Many cases of TED have duration of from several months up to about 3 years and will improve spontaneously or with the aid of treatment depending on the severity. Studies of TED have shown that Graves' patients who smoke more often experience TED or cases that are more severe.

CHAPTER FOUR

Radioactive Iodine Ablation of the Thyroid

Cell Destruction of Diseased Glands

This procedure abbreviated - RAI is performed by giving a patient an oral dose of radioactive iodine, which causes thyroid tissue death to cease its hyper-functioning.

RAI is the most commonly performed treatment for resolving cases of severe hyperthyroidism. Most people with Graves' disease, the most common cause of an overactive thyroid, are recommended for this procedure if medications fail to sufficiently slow-down an over-producing gland.

Patients with papillary or follicular thyroid cancer may also be referred for this procedure, following surgical removal of their glands (total thyroidectomy), to eradicate any remaining thyroid cells that can potentially contain malignancy.

How Does RAI Work?

The goal of RAI includes the following desired results:

• to destroy and eradicate all thyroid tissue and/or malignant cells in the body

• to stop the natural thyroid hormone production in the gland

• to correct hyperthyroidism

• to restore normal metabolism to the body

Once a dose of radioactive iodine that is large enough to completely kill the cells in a thyroid gland has been administered, the iodine is immediately absorbed by the gland. It does this because the thyroid is dependent on iodine to manufacture thyroid hormone. Once iodine enters the body through a person's diet or by oral dosing, the gland absorbs it to regulate bodily metabolism via these hormones.

An overactive thyroid gland will absorb more iodine than a normal-functioning gland will. Patients scheduled for RAI are placed on a "no iodine diet" for two weeks or more previous to the procedure, so that the thyroid gland absorbs the radioactive iodine as completely as possible.

What is the Result?

The radioactivity in the iodine enters the cells of the gland and causes them to die. The goal of the treatment is to fully eradicate all thyroid tissue from the body, so that it ceases to produce thyroid hormone. This will correct the hyperthyroidism.

Once thyroid hormone levels begin falling to lower levels following RAI, the overactive bodily metabolism slows down from the hyperthyroid state. Several weeks following the procedure the patient's thyroid hormone levels will fall to hypothyroid levels (under-active). The resulting hypothyroidism must then be treated (usually lifelong) with thyroid hormone replacement therapy to raise bodily metabolism back to a normal level.

What are the Risks?

RAI is a safe and effective procedure in most cases; there are, however, some medical sources that state that the treatment places some patients at risk for a worsening of thyroid eye disease (inflammatory condition in the eyeballs).

Other side effects that are temporary may include the following:

- sore throat

- dry mouth

- mild nausea

- dizziness

- fatigue

Some patients will rarely also see thyroid tissue that is not fully eradicated from the body that re-grows and becomes revitalized and begins producing thyroid hormone.

If it does so at an abnormally high level as it did before the procedure, this may require that the treatment be re-administered.

Patients are also required to be quarantined from family and pets for five to seven days due to risk of exposing them to radiation that remains in the body for a period following the procedure and can be spread by close contact.

Some thyroid-treating doctors offer a choice between thyroidectomy and RAI procedures to some of patients in need of thyroid ablation/removal (depending on individual cases). Patients should become educated about both options and fully discuss them with their treating doctor so that they feel comfortable and confident about the procedure they choose to have their doctors perform.

CHAPTER FIVE

Treatment for Hashitoxicosis versus Graves' Disease

Patients with Temporary Hyperthyroidism

When Hashimoto's patients developing hypothyroidism, an under-active thyroid gland, go through "Hashitoxicosis", meaning temporary hyperthyroidism (overactive) they usually only register a slight difference in blood labs or only a mild indication of hyperthyroidism on them due to progressive hypothyroidism trying to take over. In other words, though these patients alternate between hyperthyroidism and hypothyroidism, it is temporary so that lab results of their thyroid hormone levels can at times be neutral or show only mild hyperthyroidism.

These patients may however test positive for "thyroid stimulating immunoglobulin" (TSI), the auto-antibody that typically contributes to Graves' disease (autoimmune hyperthyroidism). Once hypothyroidism does take over, they will need thyroid hormone replacement as a lifelong treatment.

With Graves' disease, it settles in long enough to register as full blown hyperthyroidism on blood lab tests of thyroid hormone levels. This plus a high elevation of TSI antibodies can point to a definitive diagnosis of Graves' disease.

Rarely, Hashimoto's and Graves' can co-exist somewhat equally in a thyroid patient, so that they don't fully transition over to one or the other and when this occurs, the treatment may be destruction or surgical removal of the thyroid. Some countries treat these type patients that waver back and forth between the two disease, with a treatment called "block and replace" in which thyroid hormone blocking drugs (anti-thyroid) are first administered, followed by thyroid hormone replacement, once hypothyroidism has been fully induced. This treatment is rarely used in the USA.

Some doctors try an anti-thyroid drug or what's called a "PTU" (propylthiouracil and Carbimazole) that slows thyroid hormone production for Graves'-hyperthyroidism and after a trial of it, will wean the patient off of it after a few months and see if the hyperthyroidism resolves.

If not, they will then opt for RAI ablation (Radio Active Iodine destruction of the thyroid gland) or a thyroidectomy (surgical removal). Many will first try a beta-blocker to see if it controls the hyperthyroid symptoms before going on to a PTU or a combination of the two.

If you are recommended for getting a thyroidectomy Vs RAI ask your doctor to go over the procedure with you (risks etc...), or to refer you to a doctor who can, so you can weigh the two options. You might also ask him about anti-thyroid medications if he feels they are another possible option in your case. In short, I would say overt hyperthyroidism on blood lab test results definitely points to Graves' disease. It is not that unusual for offspring of autoimmune thyroid disease parents to develop one or the other because the two diseases (Hashimoto's thyroiditis and Graves' disease) are more closely related than most people realize.

CHAPTER SIX

Why Doctors Sometimes Delay Treatment for Hashimoto's Thyroiditis

Problems with Hashitoxicosis

I created the article following below, from a response I wrote to a fellow thyroid patient experiencing severe anxiety symptoms with their Hashimoto's thyroiditis. I commented on this aspect of their thyroid disease case in the reply that follows.

My Reply:

Sometimes doctors are cautious about starting treatment due to the fact that if they treat when your thyroid hormones are fluctuating upward, which can happen earlier into the onset of Hashimoto's, they could cause you thyrotoxicity (hyperthyroidism). This would make anxiety symptoms even worse. This fluctuation back and forth between hyper (overactive) and hypo (under active) thyroid levels is common with autoimmune thyroiditis. When hyperthyroid phases are severe, it's called "Hashitoxicosis", so in my opinion, the doctor is wise in monitoring your case.

Hyperthyroidism - The Best Darn Complete Look

He'll likely do this for while longer before starting you on thyroid hormone replacement. He likely will be blood retesting your levels at about 3-month intervals or so.

As far as treatment for anxiety symptoms, mine too were severe early into the onset of Hashimoto's thyroiditis and I personally used as-needed anti-anxiety drugs (like Xanax) but I did not use them for longer than a couple of months at a time and usually took half-doses rather than full ones. These type drugs (benzodiazepines) can be addictive and is why they should be taken with some caution. This is just an added option I would mention.

Also, you are absolutely right in that research studies state that Hashimoto's thyroiditis causes anxiety symptoms but strangely there are doctors who do not have knowledge of that fact and will tell patients that the anxiety is not thyroid-related. In addition to medical studies, thousands of patients on forums, message boards and blogs attesting to having anxiety symptoms with Hashimoto's can't all be wrong!

This is just lay-opinion but I would try low dose, as-needed anti-anxiety meds before accepting a prescription for the permanent daily-dosing type, such as SSRI antidepressants. There's nothing wrong with these and they can be greatly helpful when needed but your thyroiditis flares causing anxiety may diminish over a few months or even within a few weeks time, so starting a permanent regimen drug might be an over-kill so-to-speak at this point of observing your case. Certainly if emotional symptoms are severe or overwhelming and an as-needed drug is not helping enough, therapy can be very beneficial, as can permanent type drugs. I would never discourage any of these things when they are proven to be necessary.

CHAPTER SEVEN

Manifestations of Thyroid Eye Disease

Autoimmune Eyeball Problems and Their Treatments

Thyroid Eye Disease more commonly affects people with hyperthyroid conditions but can also occur in hypothyroid patients with thyroid autoimmunity.

Both inflammation and build up of fluid around the eyes can cause them to protrude (exophthalmos) and have an exaggeratedly wide-open appearance with Thyroid Eye Disease (TED), also referred to as "thyroid orbitopathy". The eyeball can also move forward from its position within the eye socket which can become severe in some cases (proptosis).

Patients with TED can experience dryness, redness and irritation within their eyes. A feeling of pressure and grittiness in the eyes can also occur, as well as difficulty with fully closing the eyelids. Treatments are available for this condition associated with cases of thyroid autoimmunity (diseases caused by thyroid antibodies).

Graves' Ophthalmopathy

Medical sources state that Graves' Ophthalmopathy is clinically apparent to varied degrees in up to 50% of Graves' disease patients, although other medical sources state that up to 80% of Graves' patients experience some type of eye symptoms as listed previously. While Graves' is the autoimmune cause of thyrotoxicity, also referred to as "hyperthyroidism" TED can occur in approximately 10% of patients with the auto-antibodies that cause Grave's but whose thyroid hormone levels are euthyroid, meaning within normal values. Only about 2% of Hashimoto's thyroiditis patients (those with autoimmune hypothyroidism) are affected by TED.

Optic Neuropathy

The optic nerves in the eyes of TED patients can also become affected due to their becoming compressed as a result of pressure from tissue-swelling in and around the eyeballs (orbital areas). With this condition that can be present with TED, a patient may experience pain, inability to see colors and/or partial loss of vision which will affect one or both eyes.

Nerve cell damage may occur with optic neuropathy and eventual blindness is possible if treatment for TED is delayed.

The Role of Myxedema in TED

Myxedema is a term meaning tissues in the body are retaining fluid (edema) and a build-up of mucin (mucus) will cause a thickening of the skin in areas of the body, or what is also referred to as "pretibialmucinosis". The condition is often present in autoimmune thyroid disease patients who are experiencing TED. Areas on the face can become swollen for example and will have a puffy appearance. The deep tissues around the eyes can also become swollen as well as tissues behind the eyes. This causes less area in the eye-sockets for movement and to retain the orbital position of the eyes, causing them to be pushed forward and to protrude.

Treatments for TED

The first line of treatment when TED is diagnosed is to correct any thyroid hormone imbalance that might be present if it is not already being done.

In cases when thyroid autoimmunity is the cause of hyperthyroidism, patients may need to have their thyroid glands removed. Some medical research studies state that surgical removal of the gland (thyroidectomy) may be a better choice than destruction of the gland by radioactive iodine (ablation) because of the risk the latter mentioned procedure may present to some patients with TED, in worsening the condition.

The following list of treatments may also be administered individually or in combination as determined by a treating physician.

• Prescription eye drops for added lubrication to help prevent dryness and redness.

• Corticosteroid (cortical steroid) and/or topical hydrocortisone to reduce inflammation in the eyes and in tissues surrounding the eyes.

• Radiotherapy or Decompression Surgery (possibly both) to reduce pressure in the eyeballs and to prevent potential damage to them.

- Surgery for lengthening the eyelids that do not fully cover the eyes due to protrusion of them.

- TED patients who are smokers can benefit by quitting due to chemicals in cigarettes that cause inflammation in the eyes and may also be a recommendation by their doctors.

CHAPTER EIGHT

Symptoms and Manifestations of Thyroid Storm

The Hyperthyroid Condition Requiring Emergency Care

Thyroid Storm is a condition in which a thyroid patient experiences sudden, severe hyperthyroidism that requires emergency treatment to prevent injury or death.

This disorder of extremely severe hyperthyroid symptoms is rare but due to its potential to cause bodily injury through damage to organs and possible coma or death, all thyroid patients should have general knowledge about signs and symptoms of Thyroid Storm.

Symptoms

The symptoms of Thyroid Storm will occur suddenly and with extreme force. They are the symptoms of hyperthyroidism but some of the manifestations of the condition are not typical of common overactive thyroid conditions.

The general symptoms of severe hyperthyroidism include very rapid heart (tachycardia), extreme nervousness and anxiety, chronic diarrhea, uncontrollable energy, severe hypertension and muscle weakness.

The non-typical symptoms of Thyroid Storm that occur with other severe hyperthyroid symptoms include mental confusion, psychosis (hallucinations and delusions), severe vomiting, unusual behaviors, a sudden high fever, heart arrhythmias that can progress to cardiac arrest and fainting spells. These less common symptoms are likely the ones that would point to something beyond a phase of typical hyperthyroidism. When these signs and symptoms appear, the patient should be taken into emergency medical care immediately, to prevent coma and/or death from occurring.

Is Thyroid Storm Exclusive to Hyperthyroid Patients?

No, the condition can also occur in hypothyroid patients although it is more common in those with hyperthyroidism, especially the autoimmune-caused type called Graves' disease.

Patients with hypothyroidism caused by Hashimoto's (autoimmune thyroiditis) have also been known to experience Thyroid Storm and those patients who experience intermittent phases of hyperthyroidism referred to as "Hashitoxicosis" are at higher risk for having a Thyroid Storm.

Causes and Triggers

When Thyroid Storm occurs, the T3 and T4 thyroid hormones elevate to very high levels, causing severe thyrotoxicity (toxic levels). Graves' disease patients and others who are being treated for hyperthyroidism can experience Thyroid Storm if they suffer a heart attack or a severe infection in their bodies.

Any traumatic experience can result in this condition of severe hyperthyroidism, including accidents that cause severe physical trauma. Patients treated for hypothyroidism can experience the condition, if they are given excessively high levels of thyroid hormone replacement that causes their T4 and/or T3 levels to elevate far above normal values.

Treatments

The treatments for Thyroid Storm include those that are typical for treating hyperthyroidism but in this case the drugs that are administered must be done at higher doses until symptoms are brought under control. If a hyperthyroid patient has already received treatments to shut down their own thyroid hormone production (thyroid removal) and they are taking thyroid hormone therapy, the replacement hormone must be discontinued while treatment is given.

The treating physician will increase or begin administering levels of anti-thyroid drugs (to reduce thyroid hormone levels) and beta-blocker medications that calm hypertensive and cardiac arrhythmia symptoms. Anti-inflammatory drugs may also be needed to reduce inflammation and fever levels. This may include powerful corticosteroids (steroid anti-inflammatory) and/or over-the-counter drugs that reduce inflammation. Patients are closely monitored until symptoms of Thyroid Storm have diminished and there is no danger of relapse.

CHAPTER NINE

Support for Struggling Thyroid Patients

Two Reasons Why Information and Support Resources are Important

1. Newly diagnosed thyroid patients often express the fact that despite quality treatment for thyroid disease, their doctors do not have the ability due to time-constraints, to fully inform them about their disease/disorder. Most patients feel a great need to understand what is happening to them (self-education) because the unknown aspects of thyroid problems can create fear and frustration in many patients.

2. Thyroid patients experience serious bouts of emotional issues from thyroid disease (anxiety and/or depression) and from the realities of experiencing the onset of a disease that will affect them, for the rest of their lives. A source of emotional support, such as a doctor, is not available to a patient, at any time a need might arise but only for a few minutes, at office visits that are relatively infrequent.

Patients can feel very alone with their disease and even those closest to them, may be at a loss for knowing how to support and comfort them. The facts addressed in these two points alone help to point out the purpose and importance for the availability of information and support resources, that can be shared between thyroid patients. Fellow-patients can often relate better to each other than they can to their own healthy family members.

It is unfortunate when patients are told that they should not look into support resources online because they "might be led astray with wrong information" and that they should somehow rely solely on their doctor, not only for treatment but also for needed, general education about their disease and the often-needed support for coping with it.

Getting these needs met by a treating doctor is simply not possible in most cases, unless a patient's spouse or close relative is a doctor. In the case of a patient who doesn't especially feel the need for information and support, it wouldn't be necessary to begin with but for many patients it can actually mean survival if they are seriously affected by their disease.

It is sometimes forgotten that complications from thyroid disease can include things such as Thyroid Eye Disease, Obstructive Goiters, chronic mood disorders and Thyroid Storm (potentially life threatening). Most thyroid patients have the common sense to learn from reputable sources when doing an online search about their disease and to the compare information they find with other reliable sources, so that it is confirmed. At many thyroid disease forums and message boards for example, patients share general information that can be confirmed by reputable source-links, plus they can offer support that comes from fellow-patient experience.

To deny patients this type help, for fear of them being led astray by incorrect information etc..., could mean tremendous lost opportunities for patients who have serious struggles coping with their thyroid disease.

CHAPTER TEN

Coping with Thyroid Disease

Methods for Dealing with a Lifetime Health Disorder

Educate Yourself about your Thyroid Disorder

Being newly diagnosed with a thyroid disease or disorder can be concerning and can sometimes create more anxiety in a person when they feel less informed about what is happening to them. Doctors do not always have enough time to thoroughly educate their patients about their diagnosis due to having large numbers of patients to treat as mentioned previously. Some doctors help educate their patients by providing them with informative brochures about their thyroid conditions.

In addition to information your doctor provides, you can also search online for information that will help generally educate you. Reputable and reliable sources are a great way to become better informed about symptoms, treatment and any risks for developing other related problems from your thyroid disorder.

Some of the better thyroid information sources include the AACE (American Association of Clinical Endocrinologists), MedLinePlus (National Institutes of Health), WebMD and the ATA (American Thyroid Association).

Join Fellow Patient Thyroid Forums and Support Groups

You can get connected to other thyroid patients by joining forums and groups that offer support to thyroid patients. Many of these forums are volunteer and non-profit. Others do make money from ad space they sell or share but many times this is to help run the forum or group they moderate or administrate and to cover any expenses.

By corresponding with other thyroid patients through these types of resources, you can hear their personal stories and possibly relate-to many of the things they may struggle with in regard to symptoms. You may also hear pointers for getting the best possible treatment for optimal recovery of your health and a better quality of life. There are a number of thyroid forums available, but two of the more reputable are the MedHelp International and HealthBoards thyroid disease forums.

Be Proactive in your Treatment and become a Partner with your Doctor

This simply means you are advocating representing yourself in getting the best possible treatment for your thyroid disease from your doctor. This is better accomplished by first becoming educated about your thyroid disease as mentioned in step one above. A doctor must hear as much as they can from their patient because we are the only person who can let him know how well our treatment is relieving our symptoms.

Doctors are also usually open to suggestions from patients who may feel they need a certain test run to better evaluate how well their treatment is going or in suggesting a change in the dose-level of a medication they are receiving. Of course this type partnering needs to be done in balance so that your doctor doesn't feel that you are not placing trust in him in administering proper treatment. Your goal is simply to help him know how your treatment is going and what you would reasonably like to see accomplished for you over time.

Help to Educate other Thyroid Patients

By referring fellow patients to helpful resources you have received a benefit from and by sharing your personal story you can help to educate them. Sharing the same type of support you have received can serve as a type of therapy in your own continued coping as well. Some thyroid patients, such as me, will begin to compose articles in contributing toward fellow patient education by helping share helpful and general information.

This type of help is sometimes referred to as "Thyroid Patient Advocacy" because the advocate helping fellow patients is also a thyroid patient. Some patients relate better to those who are going through the same or similar experience than they can to their healthy family members or even their own doctors. Doctors can be excellent at treating thyroid diseases, but when it comes to support and coping, fellow patients can sometimes be the best source.

If you are a struggling or a newly diagnosed thyroid patient, consider searching online for helpful information, support and sources that can help you better-cope and regain a better quality of life.

It is my hope that this ebook has been a resource that has already contributed toward that goal and I extend my sincere appreciation and best wishes to each reader!

(END)

CPSIA information can be obtained at www.ICGtesting.com
Printed in the USA
LVOW01s0305040615

441050LV00022B/482/P